HEALTHY PLATES, SLIMMER YOU

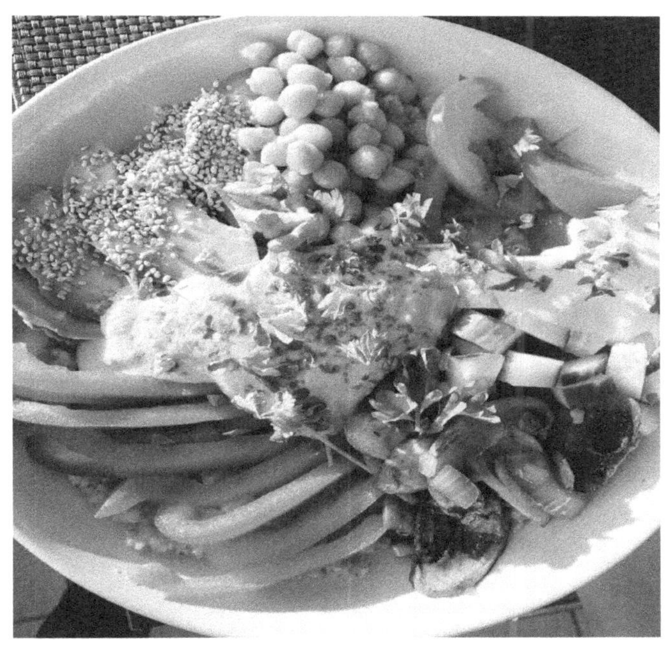

*Easy And Nutritious Meal Plan
For Sustainable Weight Loss*

Ursula Tom

TABLE OF CONTENT

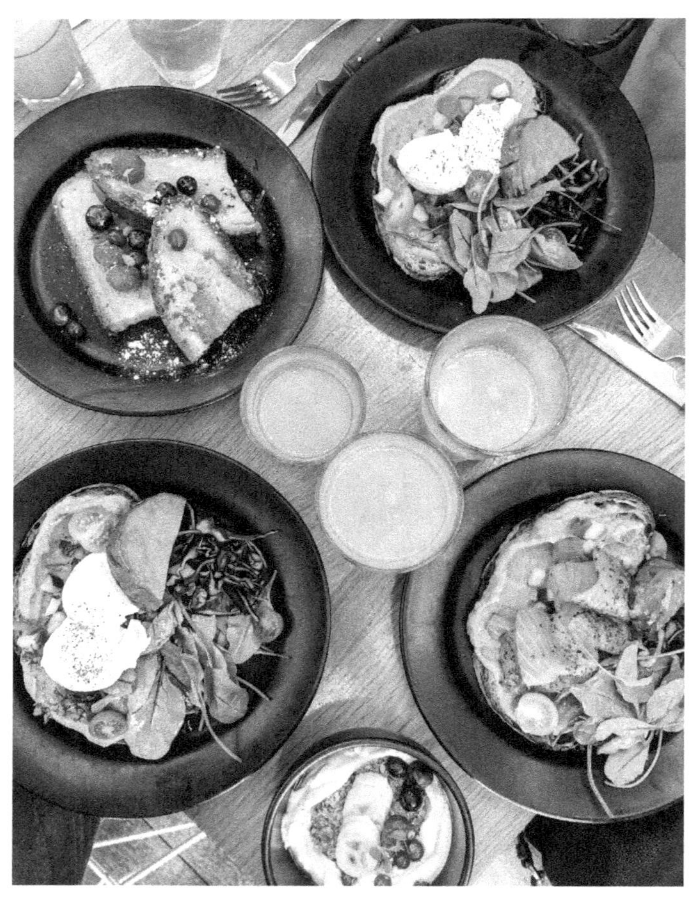

INTRODUCTION

In the relentless pursuit of well-being, the quest for a simple and healthy weight loss meal plan has become a cornerstone for individuals seeking sustainable and transformative lifestyle changes. In a world inundated with fad diets and quick fixes, the essence of a practical and nourishing meal plan is paramount.

At its core, a simple and healthy weight loss meal plan is a blueprint for achieving and maintaining a balanced physique without resorting to extremes. It champions the idea that wellness is not synonymous with deprivation but rather a harmonious integration of nutrient-dense foods that nurture the body and mind.

The allure of simplicity lies in its accessibility and sustainability. This meal plan is designed to demystify the complexities of nutrition, offering a straightforward approach that can be seamlessly woven into the fabric of daily life. By focusing on whole, minimally processed foods, individuals can forge a path towards weight loss that is both realistic and enduring.

The health-conscious journey is not just about shedding pounds; it's about cultivating a lifestyle that fosters vitality and longevity. A well-crafted meal plan recognizes the intricate interplay between various food groups, ensuring an ample supply of essential nutrients while steering clear of empty calories and harmful additives.

This introduction heralds the advent of a holistic approach to weight loss—one that embraces the joy of eating, the celebration of diverse flavors, and the empowerment of individuals to make informed choices. As we embark on this journey together, let the guiding principles of simplicity, balance, and nourishment illuminate the path to a healthier, more vibrant future.

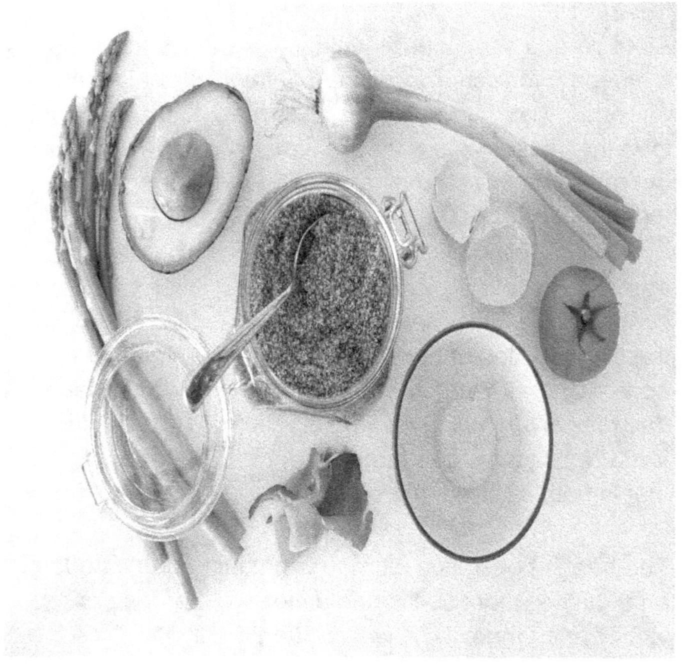

CHAPTER ONE

A meal plan for weight loss serves as a strategic tool to help individuals achieve their weight loss goals in a healthy and sustainable manner.

The purpose and importance of a meal plan and healthy eating in the context of weight loss are closely interconnected and contribute significantly to the success and sustainability of weight loss efforts. Here's an overview:

Purpose of a Meal Plan for Weight Loss:

Caloric Control:
 A meal plan helps control calorie intake by outlining specific portions and food choices. This is essential for creating a caloric deficit, which is fundamental to weight loss.
Nutrient Balance:
 A well-designed meal plan ensures a balanced intake of macronutrients (carbohydrates, proteins, fats) and micronutrients (vitamins and minerals). This balance is crucial for overall health and to prevent nutritional deficiencies during weight loss.
Portion Management:
By specifying portion sizes, a meal plan assists in managing portion control, preventing overeating, and helping individuals become more aware of appropriate serving sizes.
Meal Timing:
Planning meals and snacks throughout the day helps regulate blood sugar levels, preventing extreme hunger and reducing the likelihood of unhealthy food choices.
Adherence and Consistency:

Following a meal plan provides structure and routine, making it easier for individuals to adhere to their weight loss goals consistently over time.
Education and Awareness:
Creating a meal plan involves learning about the nutritional content of foods and making informed choices. This education promotes awareness and empowers individuals to make healthier decisions independently.

Importance of Healthy Eating for Weight Loss:

Sustainable Weight Loss:
Healthy eating promotes a sustainable approach to weight loss by emphasizing long-term lifestyle changes rather than short-term, restrictive diets. This approach is more likely to produce long-lasting results.
Nutrient-Dense Choices:
Choosing nutrient-dense foods ensures that the body receives essential nutrients while minimizing empty calories. This is crucial for supporting overall health and well-being during the weight loss journey.

Preservation of Muscle Mass:
Adequate protein intake, a component of healthy eating, helps preserve lean muscle mass. This is important for maintaining metabolic rate and ensuring that weight loss comes from fat rather than muscle.
Energy Levels and Exercise Performance:
A balanced and nutritious diet provides the energy needed for physical activity. It supports exercise performance, which is a key component of many weight loss plans.

Improved Digestive Health:
A diet rich in fiber, found in fruits, vegetables, and whole grains, promotes good digestive health. This can alleviate bloating and contribute to a sense of well-being during weight loss.
Mindful Eating:
Healthy eating encourages mindful habits, such as paying attention to hunger and fullness cues. This can reduce emotional or impulsive eating, which may hinder weight loss progress.
Reduced Risk of Nutrient Deficiencies:
Focusing on a variety of nutrient-dense foods helps prevent nutrient deficiencies, which could arise during restrictive or imbalanced diets.
Positive Impact on Mental Health:
Nutrient-rich foods have been associated with improved mood and cognitive function. A positive mental state can enhance motivation and adherence to weight loss goals.

A well-crafted meal plan, combined with healthy eating practices, is a powerful strategy for effective and sustainable weight loss. It addresses both the quantitative and qualitative aspects of nutrition, promoting overall health while helping individuals achieve their weight loss objectives.

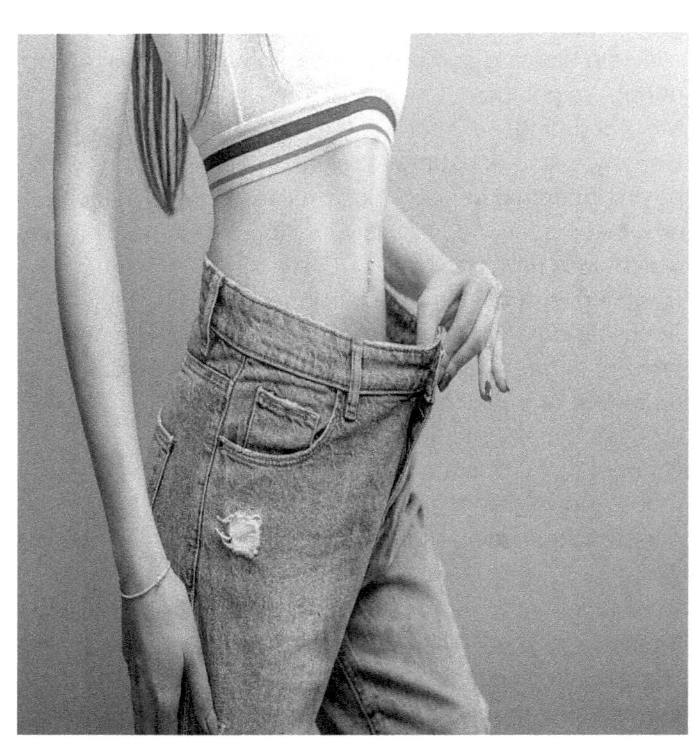

CHAPTER TWO

UNDERSTANDING NUTRITION

MACRONUTRIENTS

Macronutrients are the major nutrients that our bodies need in relatively large amounts to function properly. The three main macronutrients are: carbohydrates, proteins, and fats. Understanding each of these macronutrients is crucial for making informed dietary choices. Let's examine each macronutrient in more detail:

Carbohydrates:

Role: Carbohydrates are the body's primary source of energy. They provide fuel for various bodily functions, especially the brain and muscles.

Sources: Found in grains (bread, rice, pasta), fruits, vegetables, legumes, and dairy products.

- Types:

Simple carbohydrates: Quickly digested sugars found in fruits, candy, and sugary drinks.

Complex carbohydrates: Longer chains of sugars found in whole grains, vegetables, and legumes, providing sustained energy.

Proteins:

Role: Proteins are essential for building and repairing tissues, making enzymes and hormones, and supporting immune function.

Sources: Found in meat, poultry, fish, eggs, dairy products, legumes, nuts, and seeds.

Amino Acids: Proteins are composed of amino acids, some of which are essential and must be obtained from the diet.

- Fats:

Role: Fats play a crucial role in energy storage, cushioning organs, absorbing fat-soluble vitamins (A, D, E, K), and contributing to cell structure.

Sources: Found in oils, butter, avocados, nuts, seeds, fatty fish, and dairy products.   Types:

Saturated fats: Found in animal products and some tropical oils; should be consumed in moderation.

Unsaturated fats: Monounsaturated (olive oil, avocados) and polyunsaturated (omega-3 and omega-6 fatty acids in fish, flaxseeds, and walnuts) are considered healthier options.

UNDERSTANDING MACRONUTRIENTS IN BALANCED DIET

Understanding macronutrients in the context of a balanced diet is essential. Here are some key points:

Caloric Intake: Each macronutrient provides a certain number of calories per gram:

- Carbohydrates: 4 calories per gram
- Proteins: 4 calories per gram
- Fats: 9 calories per gram

Balanced Diet: A balanced diet typically includes a mix of carbohydrates, proteins, and fats in appropriate proportions. The specific ratio may vary based on individual health goals, such as weight loss, muscle gain, or maintenance.

Individual Needs: The ideal macronutrient distribution varies among individuals based on factors such as age, gender, activity level, and health status. Customizing macronutrient intake can optimize performance and health.

Timing: Distributing macronutrients throughout the day supports energy levels and muscle recovery. For example, consuming a combination of carbohydrates and proteins post-exercise aids in recovery.

Whole Foods: Focusing on whole, nutrient-dense foods ensures a more comprehensive intake of essential nutrients along with macronutrients.

It's important to note that while macronutrients are critical, achieving a balanced and nutritious diet involves considering micronutrients, hydration, and overall dietary patterns.

MICRONUTRIENTS

Micronutrients are essential nutrients that the body requires in smaller quantities compared to macronutrients. Despite their smaller contribution to overall caloric intake, micronutrients play crucial roles in various physiological processes and are vital for maintaining health. Here's an overview of key micronutrients and their significance:

Vitamins:

Role: Vitamins are organic compounds that support various biochemical processes in the body, including metabolism, immune function, and cell repair.

Types:

Fat-soluble vitamins: A, D, E, K; stored in the body's fatty tissues.

Water-soluble vitamins: C, B-complex (B1, B2, B3, B5, B6, B7, B9, B12); not stored in the body and need regular intake.

Sources: Found in a variety of foods, including fruits, vegetables, whole grains, dairy products, and meats.

Minerals:

Role: Minerals are inorganic elements necessary for various physiological functions, such as bone health, nerve function, and fluid balance.

Types:

Major minerals: Calcium, phosphorus, magnesium, sodium, potassium, chloride, sulfur; required in larger amounts.

Trace minerals: Iron, zinc, copper, manganese, iodine, selenium, fluoride, chromium, molybdenum; required in smaller amounts.

Sources: Obtained from a variety of foods, including dairy products, meats, nuts, seeds, vegetables, and whole grains.

Water:

Critical for hydration, nutrient transportation, temperature regulation, and overall bodily functions. Sources include water, beverages, and water-rich foods like fruits and vegetables.

Antioxidants:

Role: Protect cells from damage caused by free radicals, which are unstable molecules that can lead to cellular damage and contribute to chronic diseases.

Examples: Vitamin C, vitamin E, selenium, beta-carotene (a precursor to vitamin A).

Sources: Found in fruits, vegetables, nuts, seeds, and certain oils.

Phytonutrients:

Role: Plant compounds with potential health benefits, including antioxidant and anti-inflammatory properties.

Examples: Flavonoids, carotenoids, glucosinolates.

Sources: Abundant in fruits, vegetables, whole grains, legumes, and herbs.

Understanding micronutrients is essential for promoting optimal health and preventing deficiencies or imbalances. Here are some key considerations:

Dietary Variety: Consuming a diverse range of whole foods helps ensure an adequate intake of various vitamins and minerals.

Balanced Intake: A well-balanced diet that includes fruits, vegetables, whole grains, lean proteins, and dairy or dairy alternatives can provide a broad spectrum of micronutrients.

Bioavailability: The body's ability to absorb and use nutrients varies. Some factors, such as the form of a nutrient in food and the presence of other substances, can affect bioavailability.

Nutrient Interactions: Certain nutrients have interactions with one another that can either promote or prevent absorption. For example, vitamin C can enhance iron absorption, while calcium can inhibit iron absorption.

Supplementation: In certain situations, such as nutrient deficiencies or specific health conditions, supplementation may be recommended. However, obtaining nutrients from food is generally preferable.

Individual Needs: Individual requirements for micronutrients can vary based on factors such as age, gender, life stage, and health status.

In summary, while macronutrients provide the energy necessary for bodily functions, micronutrients play essential roles in maintaining health and preventing various diseases. A balanced and varied diet rich in nutrient-dense foods is key to ensuring an adequate intake of essential micronutrients.

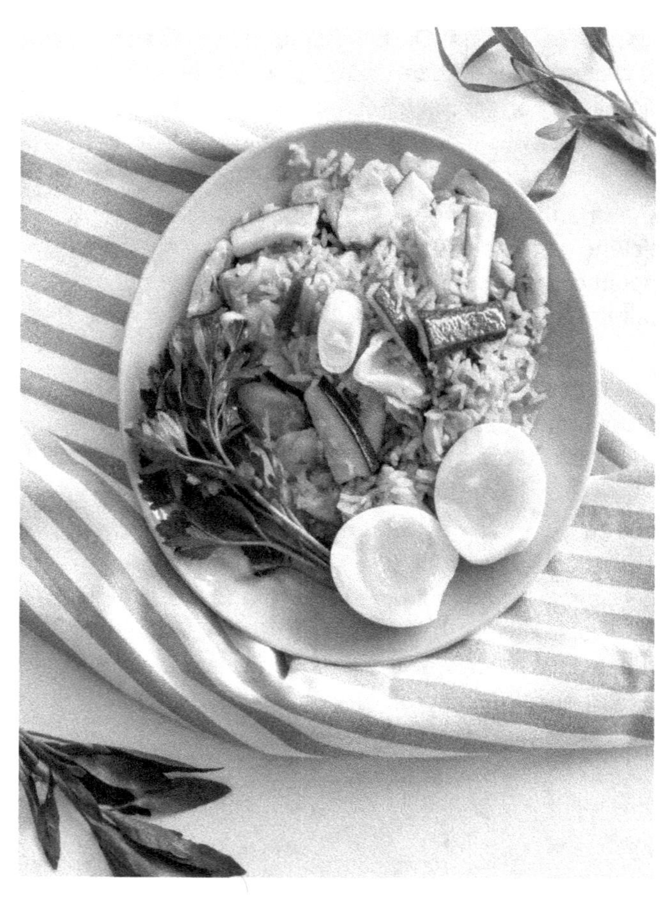

CHAPTER THREE

CREATING A BALANCED MEAL PLAN

Creating a balanced meal plan for weight loss involves incorporating a variety of nutrient-dense foods in appropriate portions while maintaining a caloric deficit. Here's a guide to help you develop a well-rounded and sustainable meal plan:

1. Determine Caloric Needs:

Determine how many calories you need each day depending on your age, gender, height, weight, and level of activity. Determine a caloric deficit for weight loss, typically ranging from 500 to 1000 calories per day for a gradual and sustainable approach.

2. Include a Variety of Food Groups:

Proteins: Include lean protein sources such as poultry, fish, lean meats, tofu, legumes, and low-fat dairy. Maintaining muscle mass while losing weight requires protein.

Carbohydrate: Complex carbohydrates can be found in whole grains, fruits, vegetables, and legumes. Choose whole grains, fruits, vegetables, and legumes for complex carbohydrates. These provide fiber, vitamins, and minerals, promoting satiety and stable blood sugar levels.

Fats: Add foods like avocados, nuts, seeds, olive oil, and fatty fish that are good sources of fat.. Moderate fat intake is important for overall health and satiety.

3. Meal Timing:

Distribute calories throughout the day with three main meals and 1-2 snacks. Eating smaller, balanced meals more frequently can help control hunger and maintain energy levels.

4. Portion Control:

Be mindful of portion sizes to avoid overeating. Use measuring tools or visual cues (e.g., palm-size for protein, fist-size for carbohydrates) to estimate portion sizes.

5. Hydration:

Stay hydrated by consuming water throughout the day. Sometimes, thirst can be mistaken for hunger. Limit sugary drinks and focus on water, herbal teas, and other low-calorie beverages.

6. Include Fiber-Rich Foods:

Incorporate plenty of fiber from fruits, vegetables, whole grains, and legumes. Fiber promotes satiety, aids digestion, and supports overall digestive health.

7. Limit Processed Foods and Added Sugars:

Minimize the intake of processed foods, sugary snacks, and beverages. Opt for whole, unprocessed foods to maximize nutrient content and support overall health.

8. Balanced Plate Approach:

Aim for a balanced plate with a mix of lean protein, whole grains, and colorful vegetables. This visual cue helps ensure a variety of nutrients in each meal.

9. Meal Prep and Planning:

Plan your meals in advance to avoid impulsive and unhealthy choices. Prepare meals and snacks in batches to have nutritious options readily available.

10. Monitor and Adjust:

Regularly assess your progress and adjust your meal plan as needed. Pay attention to how your body responds to different foods and adjust portions or food choices accordingly.

11. Incorporate Physical Activity:

Include regular physical activity as part of your weight loss plan. Exercise contributes to overall health, enhances weight loss, and supports muscle maintenance..

Remember, individual dietary needs can vary, and what works for one person may not work for another. It's important to focus on creating a sustainable and enjoyable eating plan that aligns with your lifestyle and preferences. Additionally, it's advisable to consult with a healthcare professional or registered dietitian for personalized guidance and support on your weight loss journey.

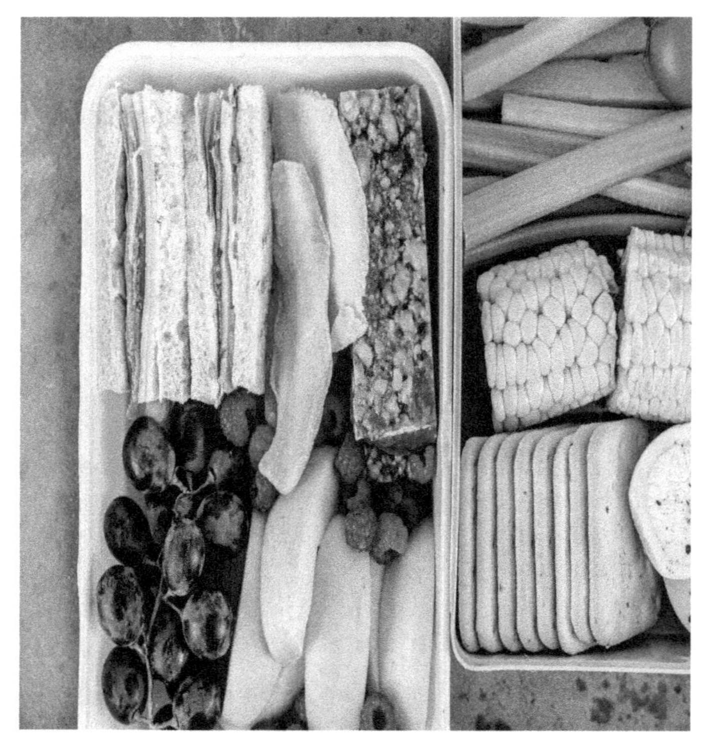

CHAPTER FOUR

SAMPLE OF MEAL IDEAS

Here's a sample of balanced meal ideas for weight loss. These meals include a mix of macronutrients (proteins, carbohydrates, and fats) and are designed to provide essential nutrients while supporting a caloric deficit. Adjust serving sizes to your unique dietary requirements and energy requirements:

Breakfast:
    Greek Yogurt Parfait:

- Greek yogurt (unsweetened)
- Fresh berries (e.g., strawberries, blueberries)
- Whole-grain granola
- Drizzle of honey or a sprinkle of chia seeds

Vegetable Omelette:
- Eggs or egg whites
- Spinach, tomatoes, bell peppers, and onions
- Feta cheese (optional)
- Whole-grain toast on the side

Snack:
    Apple with Almond Butter:
- Sliced apple
- Almond butter (or peanut butter)
- A sprinkle of cinnamon

Greek Yogurt and Berries:
- Greek yogurt

- Mixed berries (e.g., raspberries, blackberries)
- A handful of almonds or walnuts

Lunch:

Grilled Chicken Salad:
- Grilled chicken breast
- Mixed salad greens (e.g., lettuce, spinach)
- Cherry tomatoes, cucumbers, and red onions
- Balsamic vinaigrette dressing

Quinoa Bowl:
- Cooked quinoa
- Roasted vegetables (e.g., broccoli, carrots, cauliflower)
- Chickpeas
- Tahini dressing

Snack:

Carrot Sticks with Hummus:
- Carrot sticks
- Hummus for dipping

Cottage Cheese and Pineapple:
- Low-fat cottage cheese
- Fresh pineapple chunks

Dinner:

Baked Salmon with Sweet Potato and Asparagus:
- Baked salmon fillet
- Roasted sweet potato wedges
- Steamed asparagus

Vegetarian Stir-Fry:
- Tofu or tempeh

- Stir-fried mixed vegetables (e.g., broccoli, bell peppers, snap peas)
- Brown rice or cauliflower rice

Dessert (optional, in moderation):
Dark Chocolate and Berries:
- Dark chocolate squares
- Mixed berries

Beverage:
Herbal Tea or Infused Water:
- Unsweetened herbal tea or water infused with cucumber, mint, and lemon

Remember to listen to your body's hunger and fullness cues, stay hydrated, and engage in regular physical activity to support your weight loss journey. These meal ideas are just a starting point, and you can customize them based on your taste preferences and nutritional needs.

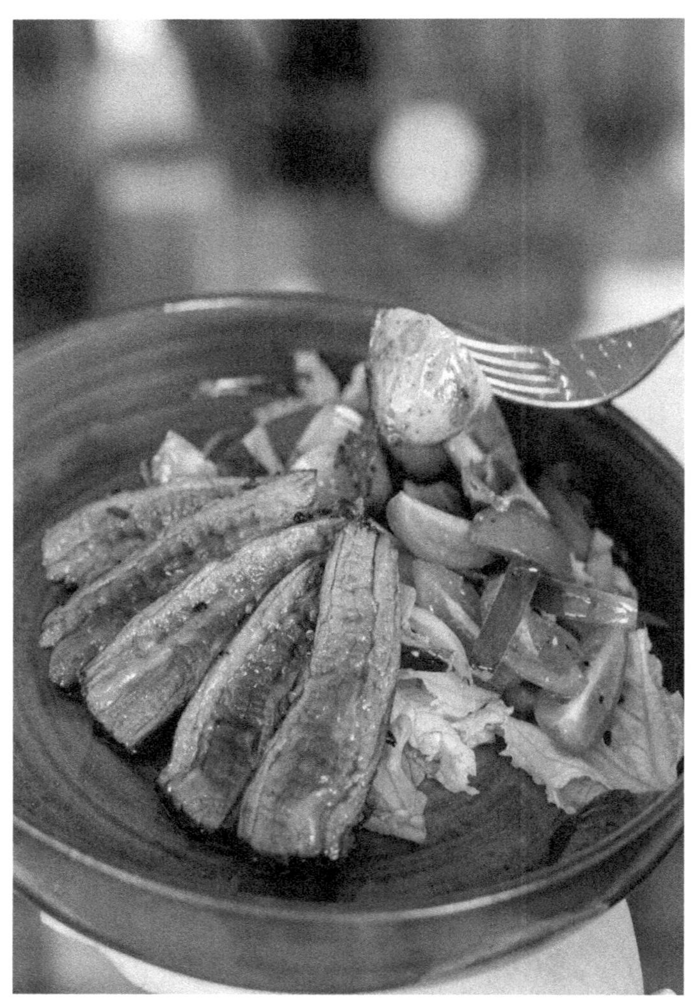

CHAPTER FIVE

COOKING TIPS FOR WEIGHT LOSS

Cooking plays a crucial role in achieving and maintaining a healthy weight. By making thoughtful choices in the kitchen, you can create delicious meals that support your weight loss goals. Here are some cooking tips for weight loss:

1. Embrace Whole Foods:

Embracing whole foods is a fundamental and highly effective approach when creating a meal plan for weight loss. Whole foods are minimally processed so that their natural fiber, nutrients, and health-promoting ingredients are retained. Incorporating these nutrient-dense foods into your diet not only supports weight loss but also provides essential nutrients for overall well-being.

Benefits of embracing whole meal:

Nutrient Density:

Whole foods are rich in essential nutrients such as vitamins, minerals, antioxidants, and fiber. These nutrients are vital for overall health and well-being, providing your body with the tools it needs to function optimally.

Satiety and Fullness:

Whole foods, particularly those high in fiber and water content, contribute to a greater sense of satiety and fullness. This can help control appetite and reduce overall calorie intake, supporting weight loss goals.

Stabilizing Blood Sugar Levels:

Whole foods, especially complex carbohydrates found in fruits, vegetables, and whole grains, have a lower glycemic index. This means they release glucose into the bloodstream more gradually, helping to stabilize blood sugar levels and reduce cravings.

Improved Digestive Health:

The fiber in whole foods supports digestive health by promoting regular bowel movements and maintaining a healthy gut microbiome. A functioning and healthy digestive system is crucial for nutrient absorption and overall well-being.

Reduced Processed Sugar and Additives:

Embracing whole foods often means reducing the intake of processed sugars, artificial additives, and preservatives. This supports weight loss by eliminating empty calories and minimizing the risk of overconsumption.

Natural Hydration:

Many whole foods, such as fruits and vegetables, have high water content, contributing to natural hydration. Proper hydration is essential for metabolism and can aid in weight loss by promoting overall health.

Enhanced Energy Levels:

Whole foods provide a steady release of energy due to their balanced combination of macronutrients. This can help prevent energy crashes and reduce the likelihood of reaching for high-calorie, sugary snacks for a quick energy boost.

Heart Health and Disease Prevention:

Whole foods, particularly those rich in omega-3 fatty acids, fiber, and antioxidants, contribute to heart health and may reduce the risk of chronic diseases. A holistic approach to health aligns with sustainable weight loss practices.

Building Healthy Habits:

Embracing whole foods promotes the development of healthy eating habits. It encourages a focus on fresh, unprocessed ingredients and cultivates a positive relationship with food.

Strategies for Embracing Healthy Foods in a Weight Loss Meal Plan:

Embracing whole foods in a weight loss meal plan is not only about counting calories but also about nourishing your body with nutrient-dense, real foods. By prioritizing whole vegetables, fruits, lean proteins, whole grains, and healthy fats, you create a foundation for sustainable weight loss while supporting your overall health and well-being. It's a holistic approach that not only aids in shedding excess pounds but also fosters a positive and lasting relationship with food. Prioritize whole, unprocessed foods like fruits, vegetables, lean proteins, whole grains, and legumes. These foods are rich in nutrients and fiber, keeping you satisfied for longer.

2. Prioritize Plant-Based Foods:

Embarking on a weight loss journey requires a thoughtful and sustainable approach to nutrition. One effective strategy gaining popularity is prioritizing plant-based foods in your meal plan. Plant-based diets are not only rich in essential nutrients but can also contribute to weight loss in a healthy and satisfying manner. Let's explore why and how you can incorporate more plant-based options into your weight loss journey.

Nutrient Density and Lower Caloric Density:

Plant-based foods, such as fruits, vegetables, legumes, nuts, and seeds, are often rich in essential vitamins, minerals, and fiber. These foods provide a high nutrient density, meaning you get more essential nutrients per calorie. Additionally, many plant-based options have lower caloric density, allowing you to consume larger portions with fewer calories, helping you stay fuller for longer.

Fiber for Satiety:

Fiber is a key component of many plant-based foods and plays a crucial role in weight loss. It promotes a feeling of fullness and helps control appetite, preventing overeating. By prioritizing plant-based sources of fiber, such as whole grains, fruits, and vegetables, you can maintain satiety throughout the day, making it easier to adhere to your calorie goals.

Rich in Antioxidants:

Plant-based foods are abundant in antioxidants, which help combat oxidative stress in the body. Antioxidants support overall health and may play a role in weight management. Including a variety of colorful fruits and vegetables in your meals ensures a diverse range of antioxidants, contributing to both your weight loss and overall well-being.

Balanced Macronutrients:

A well-planned plant-based diet can provide all the necessary macronutrients—carbohydrates, proteins, and fats—in a balanced way. Legumes, tofu, tempeh, and plant-based protein sources offer protein, while nuts, seeds, and avocados provide healthy fats. Whole grains and vegetables contribute complex carbohydrates, creating a balanced and satisfying meal.

Reduced Processed Foods and Added Sugars:

Embracing a plant-based approach often leads to a reduction in processed foods and added sugars. Whole, plant-based foods are typically less processed, providing a more wholesome and nutrient-dense option for weight loss. Minimizing your intake of processed foods can contribute to better blood sugar control and sustainable weight loss.

Environmentally Friendly:

Opting for plant-based foods not only benefits your health but also has positive effects on the environment.

Plant-based diets generally have a lower carbon footprint, making them a sustainable choice. By prioritizing plant-based options, you contribute to both personal well-being and environmental conservation.

Prioritizing plant-based foods in your weight loss meal plan can be a rewarding and sustainable approach. With a focus on nutrient-dense, fiber-rich, and whole foods, you not only support your weight loss goals but also promote overall health and well-being. Remember to diversify your plant-based choices, ensuring a well-rounded and satisfying eating experience on your journey to a healthier you.

Make fruits, vegetables, legumes, and whole grains the foundation of your meals. These plant-based foods are nutrient-dense and can be central to a successful weight loss plan.

3. Opt for Whole Grains:

Opting for whole grains in a weight loss meal plan can be a smart and healthy choice. Whole grains are rich in fiber, vitamins, minerals, and antioxidants, providing numerous health benefits. Here's how incorporating whole grains into your weight loss meal plan can be beneficial:

Fiber Content:

 Whole grains are an excellent source of dietary fiber, which helps you feel full and satisfied for longer periods. This can reduce overall calorie intake by preventing overeating and snacking between meals.

Slow Digestion:

 Whole grains take longer to digest than refined grains, leading to a slower release of glucose into the bloodstream. This helps stabilize blood sugar levels, preventing rapid spikes and crashes that can trigger cravings.

Sustained Energy:

The complex carbohydrates in whole grains provide a steady and sustained release of energy. This can help you stay active and engaged throughout the day, supporting your overall physical activity levels.

Nutrient Density:

 Whole grains contain essential nutrients such as B vitamins, iron, magnesium, and zinc. Choosing whole grains over refined grains ensures you get a more nutrient-dense option, supporting your overall health.

Digestive Health:

 The fiber in whole grains promotes a healthy digestive system by preventing constipation and supporting regular bowel movements.

When incorporating whole grains into your weight loss meal plan remember to include a variety of whole grains such as quinoa, brown rice, oats, barley, bulgur, and whole wheat in your diet. This guarantees that you receive a variety of nutrients.

Remember, weight loss is a holistic process that involves various factors, including diet, physical activity, and lifestyle choices.

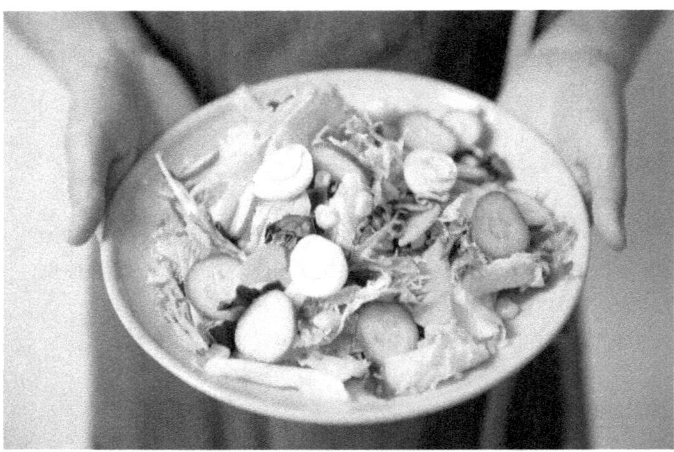

4. Portion Control:

Portion control involves managing the quantity of food you consume, which can be just as important as the quality of the food choices you make. Practicing portion control helps regulate calorie intake, prevents overeating, and supports weight loss goals. Here's an extensive exploration of the concept of portion control and strategies for implementing it in your meal plan:

Understanding Portion Control:

Caloric Awareness:

Portion control is closely linked to being aware of the caloric content of the foods you eat. It involves recognizing appropriate serving sizes to ensure you are not consuming more calories than your body needs.

Balancing Energy Intake:

Achieving and maintaining a healthy weight involves balancing the energy you consume through food with the energy your body expends through daily activities and metabolism. Portion control helps strike this balance.

Preventing Overconsumption:

Larger portion sizes can lead to overconsumption of calories, even if the foods are nutritious. Portion control prevents excessive calorie intake, which is crucial for weight loss.

Mindful Eating:

Practicing portion control encourages mindful eating. This involves being present and fully engaged with your meal, paying attention to hunger and fullness cues, and savoring each bite.

Flexibility in Food Choices:

Portion control allows for flexibility in your meal plan. You can enjoy a variety of foods in moderation without feeling deprived, making it easier to adhere to your weight loss goals.

Strategies for Portion Control:

Use Smaller Plates and Bowls:

Choose smaller dishware to create the illusion of a fuller plate. Research suggests that people tend to eat less when they use smaller plates, as it visually appears as a more satisfying portion.

Follow Serving Size Guidelines:

Familiarize yourself with recommended serving sizes for different food groups. Nutrition labels on packaged foods provide information on serving sizes and can guide you in portioning your meals.

Practice the Plate Method:

Divide your plate into sections, dedicating half to vegetables, a quarter to lean protein, and a quarter to whole grains or starchy vegetables. This method ensures a balanced and portion-controlled meal.

Weigh or Measure Portions:

Use kitchen scales or measuring cups to accurately portion foods. This can be especially helpful when cooking at home to control portion sizes and monitor caloric intake.

Learn Visual Cues:

Develop an understanding of visual cues for portion sizes. For example, a serving of meat is about the size of a deck of cards, a medium fruit is the size of a tennis ball, and a cup of cooked pasta is approximately the size of a baseball.

Eat Mindfully and Slowly:

Pay attention to your eating pace. Eating slowly and savoring each bite gives your body time to signal fullness, reducing the likelihood of overeating.

Start with Smaller Portions:

Begin with smaller portions, and only go back for seconds if you are genuinely still hungry. This prevents the temptation to eat beyond your body's satiety signals.

Be Aware of Liquid Calories:

Liquid calories from beverages like sugary drinks or high-calorie coffees can contribute significantly to your daily intake. Be mindful of these and opt for water, herbal tea, or other low-calorie alternatives.

Pack Snacks in Single Servings:

Pre-portion snacks into single-serving containers. This helps prevent mindless snacking and ensures you are aware of the quantity you are consuming.

Listen to Hunger and Fullness Cues:

Pay attention to your body's signals of hunger and fullness. Even if there is food left on your plate, you should stop eating whenever you are satisfied.

Plan and Prep Meals:

Plan your meals in advance and portion them out during meal prep. Having pre-portioned meals makes it easier to stick to your plan, especially during busy days.

Avoid Distractions:

Eat without distractions such as television or smartphones. Focusing on your meal helps you recognize when you're full and reduces the likelihood of mindless eating.

Use a Food Diary:

Keep a food diary to track your meals and portion sizes. This self-monitoring technique can enhance awareness of your eating habits and help you identify areas for improvement.

Be Mindful of Restaurant Portions:

Restaurants often serve larger portions than necessary. Consider sharing a dish with a friend, ordering appetizers as a main course, or immediately packing half of your meal to take home.

Allow for Treats in Moderation:

You can enjoy treats or indulgent foods in moderation. Rather than eliminating them entirely, practice portion control to satisfy cravings without derailing your weight loss efforts.

Practicing portion control is a fundamental aspect of a successful weight loss journey. It involves making conscious choices about the quantity of food you eat, promoting mindful eating habits, and supporting overall health and well-being. By incorporating these strategies into your meal plan, you can create a sustainable approach to weight loss that focuses on balance, awareness, and enjoyment of food.

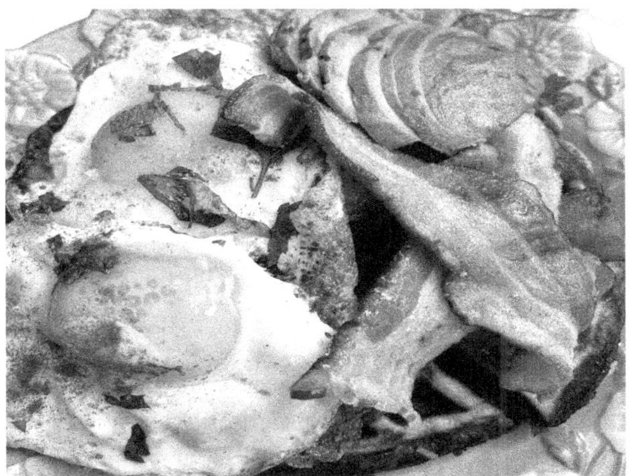

5. Choose Lean Protein Sources:

Including lean protein sources in your meal plan for weight loss is crucial for various reasons. Protein is essential for maintaining muscle mass, supporting metabolism, and promoting a feeling of fullness, which can aid in reducing overall calorie intake. When choosing protein sources for weight loss, it's beneficial to prioritize lean options to minimize saturated fat and calorie content. Here's an extensive look at the importance of lean protein and a variety of sources you can incorporate into your meal plan:

Importance of Lean Protein:

Muscle Maintenance:

Protein is vital for preserving lean muscle mass, especially during weight loss. Adequate protein intake helps your body repair and rebuild tissues, supporting overall muscle health.

Metabolism Support:

Protein has a higher thermic effect compared to fats and carbohydrates, meaning it requires more energy for digestion and absorption. This can slightly boost your metabolism, contributing to overall calorie expenditure.

Satiety and Appetite Control:

Including lean protein in meals promotes a sense of fullness and helps control appetite. This can be particularly beneficial for weight loss by reducing the likelihood of overeating and snacking between meals.

Nutrient Density:

Lean protein sources often come with additional nutrients such as vitamins and minerals, contributing to the overall nutritional quality of your diet.

Blood Sugar Regulation:

Protein helps regulate blood sugar levels by slowing down the absorption of carbohydrates. This can prevent rapid spikes and crashes in blood glucose, supporting stable energy levels.

Lean Protein Sources:

Poultry:

Skinless chicken breast and turkey breast are excellent sources of lean protein. They are versatile and can be grilled, baked, or sautéed for various dishes.

Fish:

Fatty fish like salmon and mackerel provide omega-3 fatty acids along with protein. However, for a leaner option, consider white fish such as cod or haddock.

Lean Cuts of Meat:

Opt for lean cuts of beef, such as sirloin or tenderloin, and pork, such as loin chops. Trim visible fat before cooking to reduce overall calorie content.

Eggs:

Eggs are a cost-effective and versatile source of protein. They contain essential amino acids and can be prepared in various ways, such as boiled, scrambled, or poached.

Dairy Products:

Low-fat or fat-free dairy products, such as Greek yogurt, cottage cheese, and skim milk, are rich in protein. These can be incorporated into meals, snacks, or smoothies.

Plant-Based Proteins:

Incorporate plant-based protein sources like tofu, tempeh, and edamame. These options are not only protein-rich but also provide additional nutrients like iron and calcium.

Legumes:

Beans, lentils, and chickpeas are excellent sources of plant-based protein and fiber. They can be added to salads, soups, stews, or used as a meat substitute in various dishes.

Lean Ground Meat:

When using ground meat, choose lean options such as ground turkey or lean ground beef (90% lean or higher). Drain excess fat after cooking to reduce calorie content.

Seafood:

Besides fatty fish, other seafood like shrimp, crab, and scallops are low in fat and high in protein. They can be grilled, sautéed, or added to salads for a lean protein boost.

Quinoa:

Quinoa is a unique plant-based protein source that is also a complete protein, meaning it contains all essential amino acids. It's a great alternative to grains like rice or pasta.

Seitan:

Seitan, also known as wheat gluten, is a high-protein meat substitute. It has a meaty texture and can be used in various savory dishes.

Low-Fat Cheese:

Opt for low-fat or reduced-fat cheese varieties for a protein boost without excessive saturated fat. String cheese, cottage cheese, and part-skim mozzarella are good options.

Soy Products:

Products made from soy, such as soy milk, tofu, and tempeh, are rich in protein and can be incorporated into a variety of dishes.

Strategies for Incorporating Lean Protein:

Balance Your Plate:

Aim to include a source of lean protein in each meal. This helps create a balanced plate with a combination of protein, carbohydrates, and healthy fats.

Snack Wisely:

Choose protein-rich snacks to keep you satisfied between meals. Greek yogurt, a handful of nuts, or a small serving of lean deli meat can be excellent options.

Meal Prep:

Plan and prepare meals in advance to ensure you have access to lean protein sources throughout the week. This can help you make healthier choices when time is limited.

Incorporate Variety:

Include a variety of lean protein sources in your diet to ensure you get a broad spectrum of nutrients. Rotate between different animal and plant-based options to keep meals interesting.

Watch Portion Sizes:

While lean proteins are nutritious, it's important to control portion sizes to manage calorie intake. Use visual cues or measuring tools to avoid overeating.

Experiment with Cooking Methods:

Try different cooking methods such as grilling, baking, steaming, or sautéing to enhance the flavor and texture of lean protein sources without adding excess fat.

Combine with Vegetables:

Pair lean protein sources with a variety of colorful vegetables to create satisfying and nutrient-dense meals. This adds volume and nutritional value without significantly increasing calorie content.

Incorporating lean protein sources into your meal plan for weight loss is essential for achieving your health and fitness goals. By prioritizing lean options and maintaining a balanced diet, you can support muscle maintenance, regulate appetite, and enhance overall well-being. Experiment with a variety of protein sources to keep your meals exciting and enjoyable while staying mindful of portion sizes to achieve sustainable weight loss.

5. Healthy Cooking Methods:

Choosing healthy cooking methods is crucial when you're on a meal plan for weight loss. The way you prepare your food can impact its nutritional content and overall calorie density. Opting for cooking techniques that preserve nutrients, minimize added fats, and enhance flavors without excessive calories can contribute to a successful weight loss journey. Here's an extensive exploration of healthy cooking methods to incorporate into your meal plan:

Grilling:

Grilling is a fantastic method that imparts a smoky flavor to foods without the need for excessive fats. Choose lean protein sources like chicken breast, fish, or vegetables, and marinate them in herbs and spices for added flavor.

Baking:

Baking is a dry-heat cooking method that requires little to no added fats. Use this method for proteins like chicken, fish, or tofu, and roast vegetables for a delicious and nutrient-rich side dish.

Steaming:

Steaming involves cooking food with steam, preserving its texture, color, and nutrients. Steam vegetables, fish, or even dumplings using a bamboo or metal steamer. It's a simple and efficient method that retains the natural flavors of the ingredients.

Sautéing:

Sautéing involves cooking food quickly in a small amount of oil over medium-high heat. Use heart-healthy oils like olive oil or canola oil sparingly, and incorporate a variety of colorful vegetables for added nutrients.

Broiling:

Broiling is similar to grilling but involves cooking food under high, direct heat in the oven. It's a quick method suitable for lean cuts of meat, fish, or even vegetables. Keep an eye on the cooking time to prevent burning.

Poaching:

Poaching involves gently simmering food in a liquid, typically water or broth. It's a low-fat method suitable for delicate proteins like fish or eggs. Poached chicken or salmon can be flavorful and moist.

Roasting:

Roasting allows you to cook a variety of foods in the oven at high temperatures. Use this method for vegetables, whole grains, or lean proteins. Roasting intensifies flavors without adding excessive calories.

Stir-Frying:

Stir-frying is a quick-cooking method that involves tossing small, uniformly cut pieces of food in a small amount of oil over high heat. Load up on colorful vegetables, lean protein, and use light sauces for added flavor.

Slow Cooking:

Slow cooking, such as using a crockpot or slow cooker, is a convenient way to prepare healthy meals with minimal effort. It's suitable for lean meats, beans, and vegetables, allowing flavors to meld over time without the need for added fats.

Air Frying:

Air frying uses hot air to cook food with a minimal amount of oil, resulting in a crispy texture. It's a healthier alternative to deep frying and works well for foods like sweet potato fries, chicken wings, or vegetables.

Boiling:
Boiling involves cooking food in boiling water, and it's a simple way to prepare grains, pasta, or eggs. For added nutrients, boil vegetables briefly to maintain their crispness and color.

Griddling:
Griddling involves cooking food on a flat surface, such as a griddle or non-stick pan. It's suitable for lean proteins like chicken or turkey burgers, allowing excess fat to drain away.

Microwaving:
Microwaving is a quick and convenient method that requires little to no added fats. Use it to steam vegetables, cook grains, or reheat leftovers. While not suitable for all foods, it can be a time-saving option.

By choosing techniques that preserve nutrients, limit added fats, and enhance flavors, you can create satisfying and nutritious meals. Experiment with different methods, be creative in the kitchen, and prioritize whole, unprocessed ingredients for a sustainable and enjoyable approach to healthy cooking and weight loss.

6. Limit Added Fats:

Limiting added fat is a crucial aspect of a meal plan designed for weight loss. While some fats are essential for overall health, excessive calorie intake from fats can impede weight loss goals. By making conscious choices and adopting healthy cooking and eating habits, you can reduce added fats in your diet without sacrificing flavor or nutritional value. Here's an extensive exploration of strategies to limit added fat while on a weight loss meal plan:

Choose Healthy Cooking Oils:
Opt for heart-healthy cooking oils such as olive oil, avocado oil, or canola oil. These oils are rich in monounsaturated or polyunsaturated fats, which can be beneficial for cardiovascular health when used in moderation.

Measure Cooking Oil:
Use measuring spoons or a kitchen scale to accurately measure the amount of oil you use for cooking. This helps control portion sizes and prevent excess calorie intake.

Cook with Non-Stick Cookware:
Non-stick pans and cooking sprays can reduce the need for additional fats when cooking. This is especially helpful for sautéing or frying, where minimal oil is necessary to prevent sticking.

Incorporate Healthy Fats:
Include sources of healthy fats in moderation, such as avocados, nuts, seeds, and olive oil. These fats contribute to satiety and support overall health.

Bake, Grill, or Roast Instead of Frying:
Choose baking, grilling, or roasting over frying to limit the amount of added fats in your meals. These methods can enhance flavor without the need for excessive oils.

Steam or Poach:
Use steaming or poaching methods to cook proteins like
fish or chicken. These techniques require little to no
added fat and help retain the natural flavors of the
ingredients.

Embrace Healthier Frying Alternatives:
If you enjoy the crispiness of fried foods, consider
healthier alternatives like air frying. Air fryers use hot air
circulation to cook food with minimal oil, resulting in a
lighter version of your favorite fried dishes.

Limit Butter and Margarine:
Use butter and margarine sparingly. Consider
alternatives like olive oil or avocado spread for a
healthier fat source. When using butter, opt for small
amounts or try whipped butter to spread over a larger
surface.

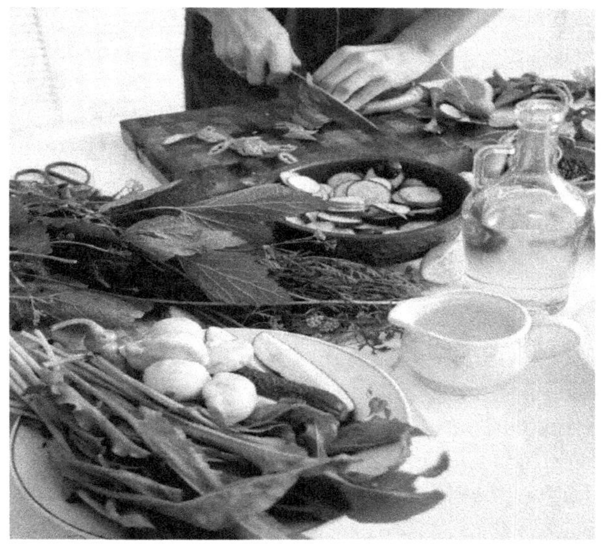

7. Load Up on Vegetables:

Loading up on vegetables is a highly effective strategy for anyone on a weight loss meal plan. Vegetables are nutrient-dense, low in calories, and high in fiber, making them a valuable addition to your diet. They provide essential vitamins, minerals, antioxidants, and fiber that contribute to overall health while helping you feel full and satisfied. Here's an extensive exploration of the benefits of incorporating a variety of vegetables into your meals for successful weight loss:

Nutrient Density:

Vitamins and Minerals: Vegetables are rich in vitamins and minerals essential for various bodily functions. These micronutrients support metabolism, immune function, and overall well-being.

Antioxidants: Antioxidants found in vegetables help combat oxidative stress in the body, potentially reducing inflammation and promoting overall health.

Fiber: Vegetables are an excellent source of dietary fiber, which is crucial for digestive health. Fiber also contributes to a feeling of fullness, reducing the likelihood of overeating.

Low Caloric Density- Weight Loss Friendly
Vegetables are low in calories compared to their volume. This means you can consume a larger quantity of vegetables for fewer calories, making them an ideal choice for weight loss.

Volume and Satiation: The high water and fiber content in vegetables contribute to their volume, promoting a feeling of satiation without excessive calorie intake.
Fiber for Satiety:

Feeling Full: Fiber adds bulk to your meals, helping you feel full and satisfied. This can be particularly beneficial for controlling portion sizes and reducing overall calorie consumption.

Blood Sugar Regulation: Fiber slows down the absorption of carbohydrates, promoting more stable blood sugar levels. This can help prevent energy crashes and reduce cravings for unhealthy snacks.
Variety of Vegetables:
Colorful Array: Aim to include a variety of colorful vegetables in your meals. Different colors often indicate

diverse nutrients, so a colorful plate ensures you get a broad spectrum of health-promoting compounds.

Leafy Greens: Leafy greens like spinach, kale, and Swiss chard are particularly nutrient-dense and low in calories. They can be incorporated into salads, smoothies, or cooked dishes for added nutrition.

c. Cruciferous Vegetables: Vegetables like broccoli, cauliflower, Brussels sprouts, and cabbage belong to the cruciferous family and are known for their health benefits. They provide fiber, vitamins, and phytochemicals.

d. Starchy Vegetables in Moderation: While starchy vegetables like sweet potatoes and carrots offer valuable nutrients, consume them in moderation to manage carbohydrate intake.

Strategies for Incorporating Vegetables:

Half Your Plate: Follow the "half your plate" rule, where at least half of your meal consists of vegetables. This ensures a nutrient-dense and low-calorie foundation for your meals.

Snack on Veggies: Choose raw vegetables like carrots, cucumber, or bell peppers as snacks. Pair them with a healthy dip like hummus for added flavor.

Vegetable-Based Soups: Enjoy vegetable-based soups as a starter or main course. Soups can be filling, hydrating, and provide an opportunity to incorporate various vegetables.

Vegetables in Breakfast: Add vegetables to your breakfast by including them in omelets, smoothies, or as a side to whole-grain options like oatmeal or quinoa.

Grilled or Roasted Vegetables: Enhance the flavor of vegetables by grilling or roasting them. This brings out their natural sweetness and adds a satisfying texture to your meals.

Vegetable Stir-Fries: Prepare vegetable stir-fries with a variety of colorful veggies. Use minimal oil and add lean proteins like tofu, chicken, or shrimp for a balanced and tasty meal.

Salads with Lean Proteins: Create hearty salads with a mix of leafy greens, colorful vegetables, lean proteins, and a healthy dressing. This can be a satisfying and nutritious meal.

Vegetable-Based Alternatives: Explore vegetable-based alternatives to traditional carbohydrates, such as zucchini noodles, cauliflower rice, or spaghetti squash. These alternatives offer more nutrients and fewer calories

Plan Your Meals: Plan your meals in advance, ensuring that vegetables play a prominent role. This helps you make intentional choices and ensures a balanced and nutritious diet.

Batch Cooking: Batch cook vegetables during meal prep to have them readily available throughout the week. This makes it easier to incorporate them into various meals.

Experiment with Recipes: Explore new recipes and cooking methods to keep your meals interesting. Be creative with seasonings and herbs to enhance the flavor of vegetables.

Make It Enjoyable: Weight loss doesn't have to be bland or restrictive. Make the process enjoyable by discovering new vegetables, trying different cooking techniques, and finding recipes that suit your taste preferences.

Loading up on vegetables is a smart and sustainable approach to weight loss. The nutrient density, fiber content, and low-calorie nature of vegetables make them a valuable addition to your meals. By incorporating a variety of colorful vegetables into your daily diet, you not only support your weight loss goals but also enhance your overall health and well-being. Experiment with different vegetables, cooking methods, and recipes to discover a variety of delicious and satisfying ways to include these nutritional powerhouses in your meal plan.

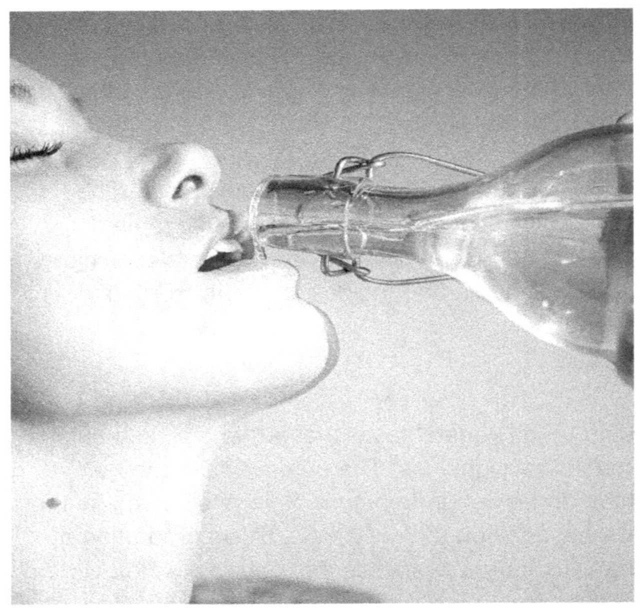

8. Hydration :

Hydration is a crucial component of any weight loss meal plan, playing a significant role in overall health and well-being. Staying adequately hydrated supports various bodily functions, including metabolism, digestion, and the elimination of waste products. Additionally, proper hydration can aid in weight loss by promoting feelings of fullness, preventing overeating, and supporting physical activity. Here's an extensive exploration of the importance of hydration and tips for maintaining optimal fluid balance while on a weight loss journey:

The Importance of Hydration:

Metabolism: Adequate hydration is essential for maintaining a healthy metabolism. Water is involved in various metabolic processes, including the breakdown of macronutrients for energy. Staying hydrated can help support your body's ability to efficiently utilize calories.

Appetite Regulation: Sometimes, dehydration is confused with hunger, which causes people to consume extra calories. Drinking water before meals can help you feel fuller, potentially reducing the likelihood of overeating.

Physical Performance: Hydration is crucial for optimal physical performance. Whether you're engaging in exercise or simply going about your daily activities, being well-hydrated supports energy levels, endurance, and overall performance.

Thermoregulation: Water is essential for controlling body temperature.. When you're physically active or in a hot environment, maintaining proper hydration helps prevent overheating and supports the body's cooling mechanisms.

Digestion and Nutrient Absorption: Water is necessary for the digestion and absorption of nutrients. It helps break down food in the digestive system and facilitates the transport of nutrients from the digestive tract into the bloodstream.

Elimination of Toxins: Hydration is essential for kidney function, aiding in the filtration and elimination of waste products from the body. Proper hydration supports the excretion of toxins through urine.

How Much Water Do You Need?

Individual Variation: The amount of water needed can vary from person to person based on factors such as age, gender, weight, physical activity level, and climate.

General Guidelines: While individual needs vary, a general guideline is to aim for about 8 cups (64 ounces) of water per day. However, some experts suggest a daily water intake of around 3.7 liters (125 ounces) for men and 2.7 liters (91 ounces) for women, including water from all sources (beverages and food).

Thirst as a Cue: Pay attention to your body's thirst signals. Thirst is a natural indicator that your body needs fluids. Additionally, the color of your urine can serve as a visual cue – light yellow to pale straw usually indicates adequate hydration.

Tips for Staying Hydrated:

Carry a Water Bottle: Throughout the day, carry a reusable water bottle with you.. Having water readily available makes it more likely that you'll stay hydrated.

Set Hydration Goals: Set daily water targets according to your personal requirements. Track your water intake to ensure you are meeting your hydration targets.

Drink Water Before Meals: Drinking a glass of water before meals can help you feel fuller and may reduce the amount of food you consume, supporting weight loss efforts.

Infuse Water with Flavor: If plain water isn't appealing, infuse it with natural flavors by adding slices of citrus fruits, berries, cucumber, or mint. This can make hydration more enjoyable without added calories.

Choose Hydrating Foods: Incorporate hydrating foods into your meals. Fruits and vegetables, such as watermelon, cucumber, celery, and oranges, have high water content and contribute to overall fluid intake.

Establish a Hydration Routine: Create a routine for drinking water throughout the day. Drink a glass of water, for instance, as soon as you wake up, before meals, and right before bed.

Monitor Hydration During Exercise: During physical activity, increase your water intake to compensate for fluid loss through sweat. Try to stay hydrated before, during, and after physical activity.

Be Mindful of Beverages: Be mindful of the calorie content in beverages. Choose water, herbal tea, or other low-calorie options over sugary drinks, sodas, or excessive amounts of fruit juices.

Limit Caffeine and Alcohol: Both caffeine and alcohol can contribute to dehydration. If consuming caffeinated or alcoholic beverages, balance them with an increased intake of water.

Listen to Your Body: Pay attention to your body's signals. If you feel thirsty, drink water. Additionally, consider factors like the climate, physical activity level, and any medications that may affect hydration needs.

Hydrate with Electrolytes: In situations where there is increased fluid loss, such as intense exercise or hot weather, consider beverages that contain electrolytes to help replenish sodium, potassium, and other essential minerals.

Signs of Dehydration:

Dark Urine: Dark yellow or amber-colored urine can be a sign of dehydration. Aim for light yellow to pale straw-colored urine as an indicator of proper hydration.

Thirst and Dry Mouth: Feeling thirsty or experiencing a dry mouth are obvious signals that your body needs more fluids.

Fatigue and Dizziness: Dehydration can cause fatigue and lightheadedness.. If you're experiencing these symptoms, consider increasing your water intake.

Headaches: Headaches can be a symptom of dehydration. Drinking water may help alleviate or prevent dehydration-related headaches.

Reduced Urination: Infrequent urination or producing very small amounts of urine may indicate dehydration. Adequate hydration typically results in regular and sufficient urine output.

Hydration is a fundamental aspect of a weight loss meal plan, supporting various physiological functions essential for overall health and well-being. By adopting mindful hydration habits, incorporating water-rich foods, and paying attention to your body's signals, you can maintain optimal fluid balance to support your weight loss journey. Stay consistent with your hydration routine, adjust intake based on individual needs, and make water a central part of your healthy lifestyle.

9. Experiment with herbs and spices:

Experimenting with herbs and spices is a flavorful and calorie-conscious way to enhance your meals while on a weight loss meal plan. By using herbs and spices, you can add depth, complexity, and richness to your dishes without relying on excessive amounts of added fats, sugars, or salt. Additionally, many herbs and spices offer potential health benefits, making them a valuable addition to your culinary repertoire. Here's an extensive exploration of how to experiment with herbs and spices to support your weight loss journey:

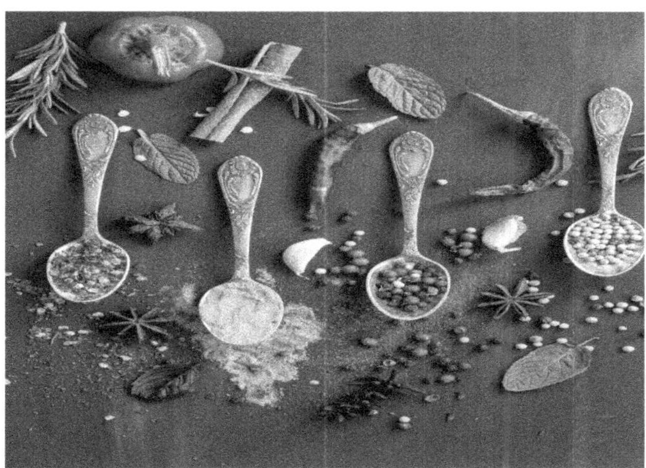

Flavor Enhancement Without Extra Calories:

Herbs and Spices vs. Condiments: Herbs and spices add flavor without the extra calories and sugar often found in condiments and sauces. By mastering the use of herbs and spices, you can create tasty meals without compromising your weight loss goals.

Satisfying the Palate: A well-seasoned dish satisfies the palate, making it more enjoyable. This satisfaction can reduce the desire for large portions and curb cravings for high-calorie, less nutritious options.

Health Benefits of Herbs and Spices:

Antioxidant Properties: Many herbs and spices are rich in antioxidants, which help combat oxidative stress in the body. Antioxidants can help improve general health and well-being.

Anti-Inflammatory Effects: Some herbs and spices have anti-inflammatory properties. Chronic inflammation is linked to various health issues, and incorporating anti-inflammatory ingredients into your meals may have positive effects.

Digestive Health: Certain herbs and spices, like ginger and mint, have been traditionally used to support digestive health. Including them in your meals can contribute to a comfortable digestive experience.

Creating Flavor Profiles:

Balancing Flavors: Learn to balance flavors using a combination of herbs and spices. Consider the interplay of sweet, sour, salty, bitter, and umami tastes to create a well-rounded and satisfying dish.

Global Cuisine Inspiration: Experiment with herbs and spices from various cuisines. Mexican, Mediterranean, Asian, and Middle Eastern cuisines, among others, offer unique flavor combinations that can elevate your meals.

Common Herbs and Spices for Weight Loss:

Cayenne Pepper: Cayenne pepper contains capsaicin, which may boost metabolism and promote fat burning. It also adds heat to dishes, enhancing flavor.

Turmeric: Turmeric contains curcumin, known for its anti-inflammatory properties. It adds a warm, earthy flavor and a golden hue to dishes.

Cinnamon: Cinnamon can add sweetness without the need for sugar. It's a great addition to breakfast items, smoothies, and desserts.

Ginger: Ginger has a spicy and slightly sweet flavor. It can be used in both sweet and savory dishes and is known for its potential digestive benefits.

Garlic: Garlic adds depth and savory flavor to dishes. It's a versatile ingredient that complements a wide range of cuisines.

Rosemary: Rosemary has a robust flavor that pairs well with roasted vegetables, lean meats, and poultry. It adds a savory and aromatic quality to dishes.

Cilantro: Cilantro contributes a fresh and citrusy flavor, often used in Mexican and Asian cuisines. It can enhance the taste of salads, salsas, and marinades.

Basil: Basil has a sweet and slightly peppery flavor. It's a staple in Mediterranean dishes and is perfect for adding freshness to salads, pasta, and sauces.

Oregano: Oregano is a versatile herb with a rich flavor. It's commonly used in Italian and Mediterranean cuisines, complementing tomato-based dishes, roasted vegetables, and grilled meats.

Paprika: There are several types of paprika, such as hot, smoked, and sweet. It adds color and depth to dishes, making it a great addition to soups, stews, and marinades.

Thyme: Thyme has a subtle earthy flavor and pairs well with a variety of dishes. It's especially popular in French and Mediterranean cuisines.

Mint: Mint adds a refreshing and cooling element to both sweet and savory dishes. It's commonly used in salads, teas, and desserts.

Practical Tips for Experimenting:

Start Small: If you're new to using herbs and spices, start with small amounts and gradually increase as you become more familiar with their flavors.

Mix and Match: Experiment with combining different herbs and spices to create unique flavor profiles. Be creative and don't be afraid to try out new combinations.

Fresh vs. Dried: While fresh herbs have a vibrant flavor, dried herbs can be more convenient and have a longer shelf life. Use fresh herbs when available, but dried herbs are a great alternative.

Consider Texture: Some herbs and spices may have a coarse texture. Consider grinding or crushing them to achieve a smoother consistency in your dishes.

Add Herbs at the End: For delicate herbs like basil and cilantro, add them at the end of the cooking process to preserve their fresh flavors.

Taste as You Go: As you cook, taste your food and adjust the seasoning.. This helps you find the right balance of flavors.

Examples of Herb and Spice Usage:

Spice-Rubbed Grilled Chicken: Create a spice rub using a mix of paprika, cayenne pepper, garlic powder, and thyme for a flavorful and calorie-friendly grilled chicken.

Turmeric-Spiced Quinoa: Add ground turmeric to quinoa along with a pinch of black pepper for a simple and nutritious side dish.

Garlic and Herb Roasted Vegetables: Toss a medley of vegetables with olive oil, minced garlic, rosemary, and thyme before roasting for a tasty and satisfying side dish.

Cinnamon-Sprinkled Sweet Potatoes: Roast sweet potato wedges with a sprinkle of cinnamon for a naturally sweet and comforting side dish.

Minty Fresh Fruit Salad: Add chopped fresh mint to a fruit salad for a burst of freshness and a hint of sweetness without the need for added sugars.

Basil and Tomato Caprese Salad: Combine fresh basil, tomatoes, and mozzarella with a drizzle of balsamic glaze for a classic and flavorful Caprese salad. Experimenting with herbs and spices is an enjoyable and beneficial approach to enhance the flavors of your meals while on a weight loss meal plan. By mastering the art of seasoning, you can create delicious and satisfying dishes without relying on excessive amounts of added fats, sugars, or salt. Embrace the diversity of herbs and spices, explore different cuisines, and make your weight loss journey a flavorful and enjoyable culinary experience.

10. Limit processed foods:

Limiting processed foods is a key strategy for those on a weight loss meal plan. Processed foods often contain excess calories, unhealthy fats, added sugars, and high levels of sodium, which can contribute to weight gain and hinder your weight loss efforts. By focusing on whole, minimally processed foods, you can enhance the nutritional quality of your diet, control calorie intake, and support overall well-being. Here's an extensive exploration of the importance of limiting processed foods and tips for adopting a whole-food approach to your meal plan:

Understanding Processed Foods:

Definition: Processed foods are those that have undergone significant changes from their original form through methods such as cooking, canning, freezing, or adding ingredients for flavor or preservation. While not all processed foods are inherently unhealthy, it's essential to differentiate between minimally processed and highly processed options.

Highly Processed Foods: Highly processed foods often contain additives, preservatives, and artificial ingredients. They are typically found in the center aisles of supermarkets and include items like sugary cereals, packaged snacks, and ready-to-eat meals.

Minimally Processed Foods: Minimally processed foods, on the other hand, undergo minimal alterations and retain much of their original nutritional content. Examples include pre-cut vegetables, whole grains, and frozen fruits without added sugars.
Benefits of Limiting Processed Foods:

Reduced Calorie Density: Whole foods tend to be less calorie-dense than processed counterparts. Focusing on these options allows you to consume satisfying portions while managing calorie intake.

Nutrient Density: Whole foods are rich in essential nutrients like vitamins, minerals, fiber, and antioxidants.

Choosing nutrient-dense options supports overall health and helps meet your body's nutritional needs.

Blood Sugar Control: Processed foods, especially those high in refined sugars and carbohydrates, can lead to rapid spikes and crashes in blood sugar levels. Whole foods with a balanced composition contribute to better blood sugar control.

Improved Digestive Health: Whole foods, particularly those high in fiber, promote healthy digestion. Fiber aids in regular bowel movements, helps maintain a healthy gut microbiome, and contributes to a feeling of fullness.

Sustained Energy Levels: Whole foods provide a steady release of energy due to their balanced nutrient composition. This sustained energy can help prevent energy crashes and reduce the likelihood of unhealthy snacking.

Lower Sodium Intake: Highly processed foods often contain excessive amounts of sodium, which can contribute to water retention and increased blood pressure. Choosing whole foods allows you to control your sodium intake more effectively.

Reduced Added Sugars and Unhealthy Fats: Limiting processed foods helps reduce the intake of added sugars, unhealthy fats, and artificial ingredients commonly found in many packaged products.

Practical Tips for Limiting Processed Foods:

Shop the Perimeter: Grocery stores typically place fresh produce, lean proteins, and dairy along the perimeter. Focus on these areas to make healthier choices and limit the temptation of highly processed items in the center aisles.

Read Food Labels: When purchasing packaged foods, read the labels carefully. Choose options with shorter ingredient lists, recognizable ingredients, and minimal added sugars and unhealthy fats.

Minimize Packaged Snacks: Opt for whole foods like fruits, vegetables, nuts, or yogurt as snacks instead of highly processed, pre-packaged options.

Cook at Home: Cooking at home allows you to have better control over the ingredients in your meals.Try out some easy recipes that call for fresh, complete ingredients..

Meal Prep: Plan and prepare meals in advance to avoid relying on convenience foods during busy times. This helps ensure that you have healthy, home-cooked options readily available.

Choose Whole Grains: Select whole grains such as brown rice, quinoa, oats, and whole wheat over refined grains. Because whole grains contain more nutrients and fiber, they make you feel fuller for longer.

Limit Sugary Beverages: Sugary drinks, including sodas and certain fruit juices, are highly processed and contribute empty calories. Choose water, herbal tea, or naturally flavored water to stay hydrated without added sugars.

Be Mindful of Sauces and Condiments: Many processed sauces and condiments can add unnecessary calories and sugars to your meals. Consider making your own or choosing options with minimal additives.

Consume Whole Fruits: Opt for whole fruits instead of fruit-flavored snacks or juices. Whole fruits provide fiber and are a more nutritious choice.

Limit Fast Food and Takeout: While convenient, fast food and takeout options are often high in calories, unhealthy fats, and sodium. Limiting these choices supports your weight loss goals.

Educate Yourself on Labels: Understand food labels and the various names for added sugars, unhealthy fats, and artificial additives. This knowledge enables you to make informed choices.

Gradual Transition:

Take Small Steps: If your current diet includes a significant amount of processed foods, consider making gradual changes. Start by incorporating more whole foods and gradually reducing your reliance on processed options.

Identify Swaps: Identify processed foods in your diet that can be easily replaced with whole, minimally processed alternatives. For example, swap sugary cereals for whole-grain oats or choose whole fruit over fruit-flavored snacks.

Explore New Recipes: Experiment with new recipes that feature whole ingredients. This can make the transition to a less processed diet more enjoyable and sustainable.

Limiting processed foods is a fundamental aspect of a successful weight loss meal plan. By focusing on whole, nutrient-dense options, you not only support your weight loss goals but also promote overall health and well-being. Be mindful of your food choices, read labels, cook at home, and gradually shift toward a diet that prioritizes the quality and freshness of ingredients. Making these changes can contribute to long-term success in achieving and maintaining a healthy weight.

11. Healthy substitutions:

Choosing healthy substitutions is a practical and sustainable approach to support weight loss goals. By making thoughtful ingredient swaps, you can reduce overall calorie intake, increase nutrient density, and create meals that are both delicious and nourishing. Here's an extensive exploration of healthy substitutions for various food categories to enhance your meal plan for weight loss:

Carbohydrates:

 Whole Grains: Substitute refined grains with whole grains: Choose brown rice, quinoa, whole wheat, or oats instead of white rice, pasta, or refined bread. Whole grains contain more fiber, vitamins, and minerals.

Vegetable Alternatives: Use vegetable noodles: Replace traditional pasta with spiralized zucchini (zoodles), sweet potato noodles, or spaghetti squash. This reduces calorie and carbohydrate intake while increasing vegetable servings.

Cauliflower Rice: Swap rice with cauliflower rice: Grated or processed cauliflower can mimic the texture of rice and is a low-carb alternative.

Legume Pasta: Choose legume-based pasta: Explore pasta made from lentils, chickpeas, or black beans for a higher protein and fiber content.

Proteins:

Lean Protein Sources: Opt for lean proteins: Choose lean cuts of meat, poultry without skin, fish, tofu, tempeh, or legumes for protein sources with lower saturated fat content.

Ground Turkey or Chicken: Substitute ground beef with lean ground turkey or chicken: This reduces the fat content while maintaining protein intake.

Greek Yogurt: Use Greek yogurt as a protein source: Instead of sugary yogurt or cream, opt for plain Greek yogurt as a base for sauces, dips, or dressings.

Cottage Cheese: Incorporate cottage cheese: Add cottage cheese to smoothies, salads, or as a topping. It's a protein-rich option with a satisfying texture.

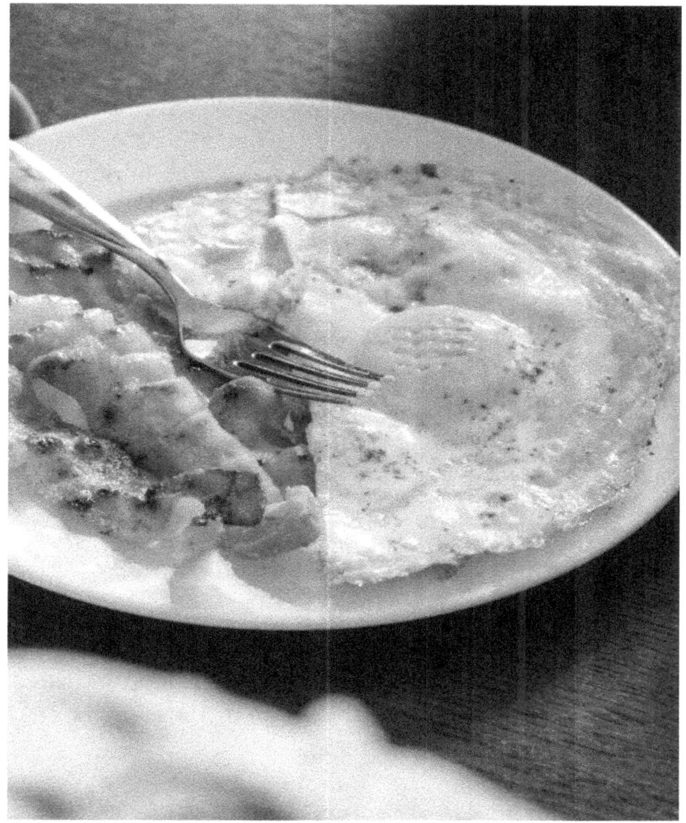

Fats and Oils:

Healthy Cooking Oils: Choose healthier cooking oils: Replace saturated fats with heart-healthy options like olive oil, avocado oil, or coconut oil in moderation.

Avocado as a Spread: Use avocado instead of butter or mayonnaise: Spread mashed avocado on toast or use it in place of mayo in sandwiches for a nutrient-rich alternative.

Nuts and Seeds: Add nuts and seeds for crunch: Instead of croutons, sprinkle chopped nuts or seeds on salads for added texture and healthy fats.

Nutritional Yeast: Opt for nutritional yeast: Use nutritional yeast as a substitute for cheese in various dishes. It provides a savory flavor without the saturated fat content.

Sweeteners:

Natural Sweeteners: Choose natural sweeteners: Replace refined sugars with options like honey, maple syrup, or agave nectar. Use these in moderation for sweetness with added nutrients.

Fresh Fruit as Sweeteners: Sweeten with fresh fruit: Use mashed bananas, applesauce, or pureed dates to add sweetness to baked goods without relying on refined sugars.

Stevia or Monk Fruit: Consider stevia or monk fruit: These natural, non-caloric sweeteners can be used as sugar substitutes in beverages or recipes.

Dairy and Dairy Alternatives:

Low-Fat or Plant-Based Milk: Choose low-fat or plant-based milk: Opt for skim milk, almond milk, soy milk, or other plant-based alternatives to reduce saturated fat content.

Low-Fat Cheese: Use reduced-fat cheese: Select cheeses with lower fat content or try nutritional yeast as a cheese alternative.

Greek Yogurt: Select Greek yogurt: Choose plain, non-fat Greek yogurt instead of full-fat versions for a protein-rich dairy option.

Snacks:

Fresh Fruit or Veggies: Snack on fresh produce: Choose fruits or vegetables as snacks instead of processed, high-calorie options.

Trail Mix with Nuts and Seeds: Make your trail mix: Create a customized trail mix with nuts, seeds, and dried fruits, avoiding the excess sugar and unhealthy fats often found in prepackaged mixes.

Air-Popped Popcorn: Opt for air-popped popcorn: Instead of buttery or caramel-coated popcorn, air-pop your kernels and season them with herbs or nutritional yeast for flavor.

Beverages:

Herbal Tea or Infused Water: Choose calorie-free beverages: Opt for herbal tea, infused water, or plain water instead of sugary drinks, sodas, or high-calorie coffee beverages.

Black Coffee: Limit additives in coffee: Drink black coffee or use a small amount of unsweetened almond milk or a natural sweetener to keep your coffee low in calories.

Coconut Water: Hydrate with coconut water: Instead of sugary sports drinks, consider coconut water for hydration without added sugars.

Baking and Cooking:

Applesauce or Greek Yogurt in Baking: Substitute in baking: Replace butter or oil with applesauce or Greek yogurt in baking recipes to reduce the overall fat content.

Whole Wheat Flour: Use whole wheat flour: Incorporate whole wheat flour instead of refined white flour for added fiber and nutrients in baked goods.

Cocoa Powder: Choose cocoa powder: Use unsweetened cocoa powder instead of chocolate chips or sweetened chocolate in recipes for a rich flavor without added sugars.

Condiments:

Homemade Dressings: Make your dressings: Prepare homemade salad dressings using olive oil, vinegar, herbs, and spices, avoiding commercial dressings high in added sugars and unhealthy fats.

Mustard or Hummus as Spreads: Use mustard or hummus: Swap mayo with mustard or hummus for sandwiches and wraps to reduce calorie and fat content.

Salsa or Pico de Gallo: Opt for salsa: Use salsa or pico de gallo instead of creamy sauces or dips for a low-calorie, flavorful alternative.

Mindful Eating:

Portion Control: Practice portion control: Be mindful of serving sizes to prevent overeating, even when making healthier substitutions.

Listen to Hunger Cues: Eat when hungry, stop when satisfied: Pay attention to your body's hunger and fullness cues, allowing you to maintain a healthy relationship with food.

Making healthy substitutions is a practical and enjoyable way to enhance your weight loss meal plan. By choosing nutrient-dense options, reducing added sugars and unhealthy fats, and incorporating a variety of whole foods, you can create meals that support your weight loss goals while nourishing your body. Experiment with these substitutions, be creative in the kitchen, and find the combinations that work best for your taste preferences and lifestyle. Remember that sustainable changes over time contribute to long-term success in achieving and maintaining a healthy weight.

12.   Be flexible:

Flexibility is a key component of a successful and sustainable meal plan for weight loss. It involves adapting your dietary approach to accommodate different situations, preferences, and unexpected challenges without abandoning your overall health goals.

Embracing flexibility in your meal plan can enhance adherence, reduce stress, and make the weight loss journey more enjoyable. Being too rigid can lead to frustration and discouragement. Flexibility allows for adjustments based on real-life situations, preventing feelings of failure if the plan deviates occasionally.

Flexibility is also crucial when attending social events or dining out. Rather than stressing over sticking to your plan, make informed choices, and focus on balance. You can compensate by adjusting your meals before or after the event.

Flexibility means eating when you're hungry and stopping when you're satisfied, rather than rigidly adhering to set meal times or portion sizes. Pay attention to your body's hunger and fullness cues.

A flexible meal plan accommodates your taste preferences and cravings. Experiment with different foods and recipes to keep meals interesting and enjoyable while still meeting your nutritional needs.

Flexibility includes recognizing that your caloric needs may vary from day to day. If you're more active on certain days, adjust your calorie intake accordingly to ensure you are fueling your body appropriately.

 Allow yourself some flexibility. Occasional treats or indulgences can be part of a healthy, balanced lifestyle. The key is moderation.

In conclusion, flexibility in a weight loss meal plan is about finding a healthy balance between structure and adaptability. It allows you to navigate the challenges of daily life while still working towards your weight loss goals. Remember, the journey is unique to each individual, and embracing flexibility can contribute to a positive and sustainable approach to nutrition and overall well-being.

13.   Track your food intake:

Tracking your food intake can be a valuable tool in a weight loss journey. It helps you become more aware of your eating habits, identifies patterns, and allows you to make informed choices. Here are some effective ways to track your food intake for weight loss:

Food Diary or Journal:

Record everything you eat and drink throughout the day, along with the amounts you consume..

Note the time of day you eat and any associated feelings or circumstances (e.g., stress, boredom, social events).

Be honest and detailed in your entries.

Use a Food Tracking App:

There are many mobile apps available that make tracking food intake convenient. Examples include MyFitnessPal, Lose It!, and Cronometer.

These apps often have extensive databases of foods, making it easier to log meals accurately.

Some apps also provide nutritional information and can sync with fitness trackers.

Nutrient Breakdown:

Track not only calories but also macronutrients (carbohydrates, proteins, and fats) to ensure a balanced diet.

Pay attention to the quality of your food choices, aiming for a variety of nutrient-dense foods.

Set Realistic Goals:

Establish realistic and achievable goals for weight loss. Aim for a gradual and sustainable rate of weight loss, such as 1-2 pounds per week.

Adjust your caloric intake according to your goals and progress.

Regular Check-Ins:

Review your food diary or app regularly to identify trends and make adjustments to your eating habits.

Celebrate your successes and learn from challenges.

14.   Stay consistent:

Consistency is essential for achieving and maintaining weight loss. Here are some key principles to help you maintain consistency in your weight loss journey:

Create a Sustainable Plan:

Develop a balanced and sustainable eating plan that you can maintain over the long term. Avoid extreme diets or drastic changes that are difficult to stick to.

Build Healthy Habits:

Focus on building healthy habits that contribute to both weight loss and overall well-being. This might include regular exercise, adequate sleep, and stress management.

Be Patient:

Weight loss is a gradual process that may not yield immediate results. Be patient and stay committed to your plan even if progress seems slow.

Track Progress:

Regularly monitor your progress, but don't solely rely on the scale. Consider other measures like changes in energy levels, fitness improvements, and changes in how your clothes fit.

Stay Consistent with Diet and Exercise:

Consistency in both your diet and exercise routine is key. Aim to make healthier food choices consistently, and incorporate regular physical activity into your routine.

Plan for Setbacks:

Understand that setbacks may happen, such as a day of overeating or missing a workout. Instead of viewing these as failures, see them as opportunities to learn and make adjustments.

Seek Support:

Share your weight loss goals with friends, family, or a support group. A support system can offer encouragement, accountability, and motivation.

Celebrate Small Wins:

No matter how small, acknowledge and celebrate your accomplishments.I. Recognize the positive changes you've made and use them as motivation to continue.

Adapt to Changes:

Be flexible and adapt to changes in your routine,
schedule, or preferences. Find alternative ways to stay
active or prepare healthy meals when faced with
obstacles.

Prioritize Self-Care:

Take care of your overall well-being, including managing
stress and getting adequate sleep. A healthy lifestyle
contributes to both weight loss and overall health.

Remember that consistency is not about perfection but
about making persistent efforts towards your goals. If
you encounter challenges or setbacks, it's okay—what
matters most is your ability to bounce back and stay
committed to your journey over time. If needed, consider
seeking guidance from healthcare professionals or a
registered dietitian to help tailor a plan that aligns with
your individual needs and lifestyle.

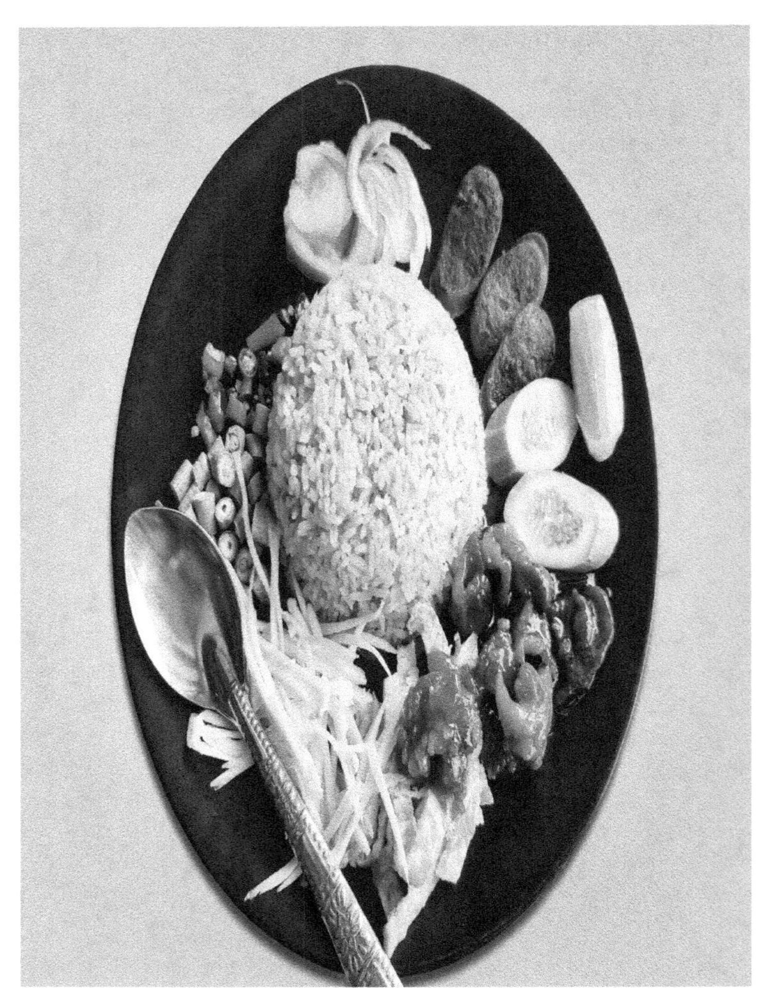

CHAPTER SIX

OVERCOMING CHALLENGES

Embarking on a weight loss meal plan can be challenging, but with determination, consistency, and the right mindset, you can overcome obstacles. Here are some common challenges people face during a weight loss journey and tips on how to overcome them:

Cravings and Hunger:

Solution: Choose nutrient-dense, high-fiber foods that keep you full longer. Include protein, healthy fats, and complex carbohydrates in each meal. Drinking water before meals can also help curb hunger.

Social Pressures:

Solution: Communicate your goals with friends and family. Choose restaurants with healthier options, and be confident in making choices that align with your plan. Surround yourself with supportive individuals who understand your commitment.

Lack of Motivation:

Solution: Set clear, achievable goals. Celebrate small victories and track your progress. Find a workout buddy or join a community for accountability and motivation.Change up your workouts to keep things interesting.

Boredom with Meals:

Solution: Experiment with new recipes and cooking methods. Incorporate a variety of colorful fruits and vegetables to make your meals visually appealing. Consider trying new cuisines to keep your taste buds engaged.

Plateaus:

A weight loss plateau refers to a period during a weight loss journey when a person's body weight stabilizes, and they experience a temporary halt or slowdown in the progress of losing weight. Despite maintaining the same diet and exercise routine that previously resulted in weight loss, the scale may stop moving or show minimal changes. Plateaus can be frustrating, but they are a common occurrence and can be addressed with the right strategies.

Solution: Reevaluate your caloric needs. It may be necessary to adjust your calorie intake by either reducing it slightly or incorporating short periods of increased calorie consumption to "reset" your metabolism.

Lack of Time:

Solution: Plan and prepare your meals in advance. Batch-cooking can save time during the week. Choose simple and quick recipes, and keep healthy snacks on hand. Make physical activity a priority by planning it into your daily schedule.

Emotional Eating:

Solution: Identify triggers for emotional eating and find alternative coping mechanisms such as going for a walk, journaling, or talking to a friend. Practice mindful eating by savoring each bite and recognizing hunger and fullness cues.

Inconsistent Results:

Solution: Weight loss is a gradual process. Focus on overall well-being rather than the scale alone. Track non-scale victories like improved energy levels, better sleep, and increased fitness. Seek the counsel of a medical expert for tailored guidance.

Lack of Support:

Solution: Surround yourself with a supportive network, whether it's friends, family, or an online community. Share your goals and seek encouragement. Consider joining fitness classes or groups to connect with like-minded individuals.

Health Issues:

Solution: Consult with a healthcare professional before starting any weight loss plan, especially if you have underlying health conditions. They can provide guidance on a safe and effective approach tailored to your individual needs.

Remember, overcoming challenges is a gradual process, and being patient with yourself is key. Long-term

success will be influenced by maintaining consistency
and adopting sustainable lifestyle adjustments.

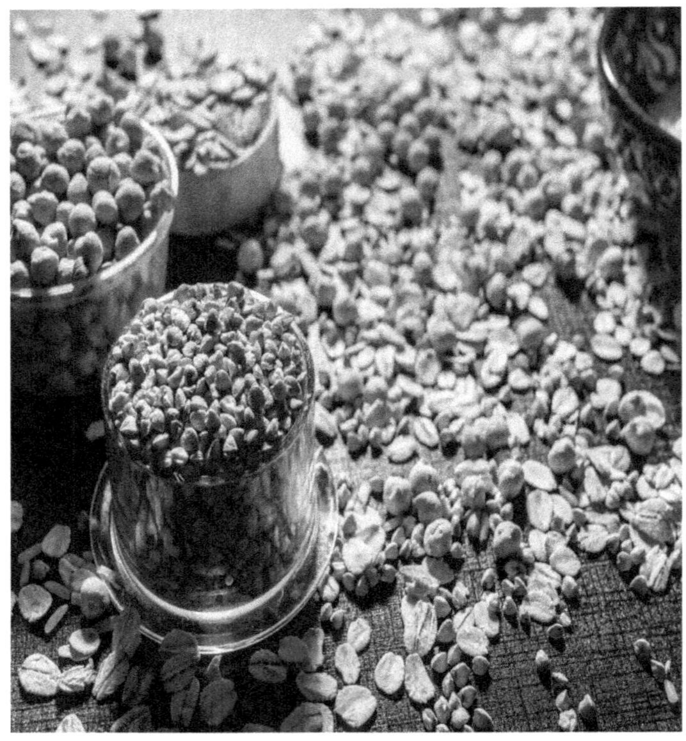

CONCLUSION

In conclusion, adopting a simple and healthy meal plan is a sustainable and effective approach to achieving weight loss goals. The key to success lies in creating a balanced and nutritious eating routine that not only supports weight loss but also promotes overall well-being. By emphasizing whole foods, incorporating a variety of nutrient-dense ingredients, and being mindful of portion sizes, individuals can embark on a journey towards healthier living.

One of the essential aspects of a successful weight loss meal plan is flexibility. Tailoring the plan to individual preferences, dietary requirements, and lifestyle constraints enhances adherence and long-term success. The inclusion of lean proteins, whole grains, fruits, vegetables, and healthy fats ensures that nutritional needs are met while providing a diverse and satisfying range of flavors.

Furthermore, staying hydrated and incorporating regular physical activity complement the dietary efforts in achieving and maintaining a healthy weight. Consistency is key, and small, sustainable changes over time contribute significantly to overall success. Celebrating non-scale victories, such as increased energy levels, improved mood, and enhanced fitness, reinforces the positive impact of a healthy meal plan beyond just the number on the scale.

It's important to approach weight loss with a positive mindset and recognize that setbacks may occur. Understanding and overcoming challenges, whether they be cravings, plateaus, or lifestyle disruptions, involves patience and a commitment to continuous improvement. Seeking support from friends, family, or a community with similar goals can provide encouragement and accountability during the journey.

In conclusion, a simple and healthy meal plan for weight loss is not just about shedding pounds; it's about fostering a sustainable and enjoyable way of eating that promotes overall health and well-being. By making informed choices, staying consistent, and embracing a balanced lifestyle, individuals can navigate their weight loss journey with confidence, ensuring that the changes made are not only effective but also lasting.